COMPACT GUIDES TO FITNESS & HEALTH

LIVE LONGER, LIVE BETTER

CONTENT PROVIDED BY MAYO CLINIC HEALTH INFORMATION

MASON CREST PUBLISHERS
Philadelphia, Pennsylvania

Live Longer, Live Better provides reliable, practical, easy-to-understand information on living a longer and healthier life. Much of the information comes directly from the experience of Mayo Clinic physicians, nurses, registered dietitians, health educators and other health care professionals. This book supplements the advice of your personal physician, whom you should consult for individual medical problems. MAYO, MAYO CLINIC, MAYO CLINIC HEALTH INFORMATION and the Mayo triple-shield logo are marks of Mayo Foundation for Medical Education and Research.

Hardcover Library Edition Published 2002

Mason Crest Publishers

370 Reed Road

Suite 302

Broomall, PA 19008-0914

(866) MCP-BOOK (toll free)

First Printing

1 2 3 4 5 6 7 8 9 10

Library of Congress Cataloging-in-Publication Data on file at the Library of Congress

ISBN 1-59084-256-1 (hc)

Printed in the United States of America

Contents

Introduction

Live longer, live better. For more than a century, medical care at Mayo Clinic has helped millions of people do just that.

But how do Mayo Clinic experts themselves grow older healthfully? To find out, doctors and other health care professionals who have helped develop Mayo Clinic books, newsletters and other health publications were asked what they do personally to improve the length and quality of their lives. Their top recommendations, along with how they personally practice this advice, are featured inside.

Some of these strategies won't come as a surprise to you. Be physically active. Don't smoke. Make your health a priority. Most of us have heard these before.

But many experts take a broader approach than just physical health. To live longer and better, according to Mayo Clinic experts, it's important to stay healthy emotionally and mentally, too. That's why some of the top recommendations listed inside include exercising your mind, investing in important relationships and staying connected to your community. You'll also learn tips on leading a full, active life after retirement.

Aging is inevitable. And nothing can guarantee you'll live longer or better. But these strategies from Mayo Clinic experts can help you put the pieces in place to make the years ahead happier and healthier.

Stay Physically Active

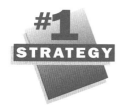

Not surprisingly, staying physically active was one of our experts' top prescriptions for a longer, healthier life — both for themselves and you.

It's easy to understand why. Even in moderate amounts, exercise can help you enjoy life and avoid diseases and conditions that many people mistakenly believe come automatically with age. And exercise doesn't have to be painful or strenuous to benefit you. Even moderately intense activities, such as a brisk walk, gardening or yardwork, can improve your health when done regularly.

You can reduce your risk of dying prematurely by almost half if you exercise every day or almost every day. Regular physical activity cuts your risk of:

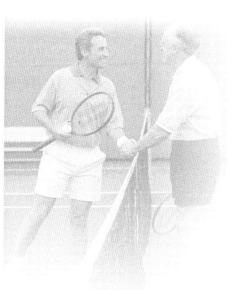

- Heart attack
- Stroke
- High blood pressure
- Diabetes
- Osteoporosis
- Depression and anxiety
- Osteoarthritis
- Falls and broken bones
- Some kinds of cancer

Exercise can be a daunting idea, especially if you're not in shape or have a hectic schedule. Here's how Mayo Clinic experts have made exercise a part of their strategies to live longer and better.

Charles Kennedy, M.D.

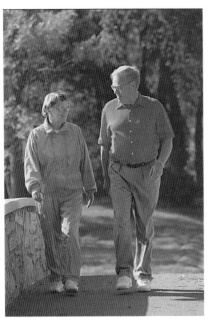

Dr. Charles Kennedy and his wife, Helen, enjoy walking together.

A 1997 hip replacement operation didn't end the commitment Charles Kennedy, M.D., has to making regular exercise a part of his life.

Although the retired internist opted to hang up his running shoes after years of enjoying road races and an occasional marathon, Dr. Kennedy simply switched gears in his exercise program. His new hip, he decided, was an opportunity to explore and enjoy other kinds of physical activity.

"I needed to make some modifications, that's all," says Dr. Kennedy, a former medical editor of the *Mayo Clinic Health Letter*.

Dr. Kennedy looked at a variety of activities and decided that swimming seemed like a good choice. It gave him a healthy aerobic workout, placed little stress on his hip, and there was a public pool at a nearby YMCA.

There was just one small problem.

"I'm not a very good swimmer," Dr. Kennedy says.

He dived into the new activity anyway, making up for his lack of swimming expertise by using a mask and snorkel. This allows him to stroke and kick without having to worry about breathing techniques.

Dr. Kennedy also made bicycling and walking a part of his routine. The walking he especially enjoys because his wife, Helen, often accompanies him.

"It's nice because it's something we can do together," he says.

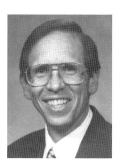

Dr. Creagan

Edward Creagan, M.D.

Edward Creagan, M.D., has always gotten plenty of exercise. The Mayo Clinic cancer specialist has been a dedicated runner for years.

But during an annual physical exam, Dr. Creagan was told he could improve his fitness routine by starting a weightlifting program for muscle strengthening. "My doctor said I was in great physical health, but I was going to start getting injured if I didn't maintain my muscle mass," Dr. Creagan says.

At his next road race, Dr. Creagan looked around and found evidence to back up his doctor's advice. He realized there were few runners left in his age group. That was all he needed to make weightlifting a part of his fitness routine.

Now Dr. Creagan works out with weights several times a week, targeting muscle groups in his arms, legs, back and abdominal areas. Although it's different than running, he enjoys both the activity and the feeling of strength it creates.

Dr. Creagan plans on lifting weights "forever," and urges others, especially older people, to do the same. Without strengthening exercises, both men and women lose about 1 percent of their muscle mass a year starting at age 30, he notes. A sensible weightlifting routine involves doing a set of 8 to 12 repetitions three times a week, but check with your doctor before starting a program.

"No matter what your age or physical fitness level, you can benefit from a weightlifting routine — as long as you begin slowly, " Dr. Creagan says.

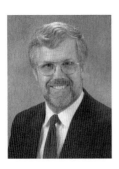

Dr. Martenson

James Martenson, M.D.

When the alarm rang at 5:30 a.m., James Martenson, M.D., found it difficult to pull back the covers and put on his jogging shoes.

"I just wasn't motivated," says the specialist in cancer radiation treatment. Then he discovered squash — the kind you play, not the kind you eat.

"Once I found something I really liked, it was no longer a case of thinking, 'How do I fit my exercise in?'" Dr. Martenson says. "I wanted to do it."

Squash, which is similar to racquetball, is a fast-paced game that's played with another person. Dr. Martenson first took it up when he was a student at the University of Washington. Now he plays three to five times a week on courts near the Mayo Clinic campus in downtown Rochester, Minnesota.

The 5:30 a.m. alarm makes sure he gets plenty of exercise before work.

"I think there is something out there for everyone that they can really enjoy, " Dr. Martenson says. "Enjoying exercise is a huge key to continuing the activity and benefiting from it."

Exercise Your Mind

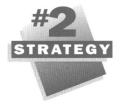

#2 STRATEGY

Just as physical activity keeps your body strong, mental activity keeps your mind sharp and agile.

If you continue to learn and challenge yourself — whether it's by learning a foreign language, switching careers or doing crossword puzzles — your brain continues to grow, literally. Regardless of your age, an active brain produces new synapses, which are connections between nerve cells that allow these cells to communicate with one another. This helps you store and retrieve information more easily, even if your "gray matter" is topped by gray hair.

While it's true that older people in general learn differently than younger people and have more difficulty with short-term memory, old age isn't an automatic slide into dementia. Numerous studies show that older people can and do learn new things — and

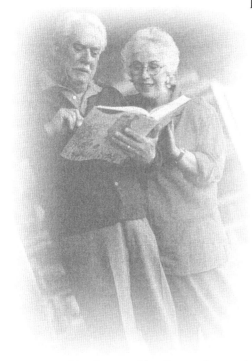

learn them well. Memory exercises and recall techniques can improve your memory and enhance your learning.

Seeking out new learning opportunities, practicing existing skills and embracing change can help you stay mentally fit no matter what your age, according to Mayo Clinic experts. On the next few pages, you'll find out how they put this advice into practice in their own lives.

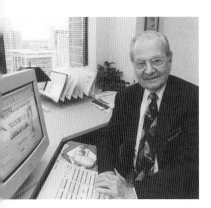

Colleagues sometimes refer to Dr. Ken Berge as "Cyberdoc" because of his role in helping pioneer the electronic information age at Mayo Clinic.

Kenneth Berge, M.D.

As one of the medical editors of MayoClinic.com, Mayo Clinic's award-winning Web site, Kenneth Berge, M.D., is helping pioneer the electronic health information age at Mayo. A retired internal medicine specialist, he reviews and develops consumer health information articles published on the site at *www.MayoClinic.com.*

When he's in Rochester, Dr. Berge works out of the editorial office. But during the Minnesota winter, when he's enjoying sunny weather down South, he works on articles and communicates with the rest of the staff via e-mail from his laptop computer.

Dr. Berge says many people his age are surprised both with his computer expertise and his willingness to work after retirement. From Dr. Berge's perspective, it's simply an intriguing way to stay in touch with medicine and stay sharp mentally.

"If you don't keep up with things, then you're going to slow down in other areas of your life," he says. "You need to have interests, no matter how old you are. Just because you're 60, 70 or 80 doesn't mean you have to roll over and give up on things."

Dr. Berge also likes demonstrating to others of his generation that computers aren't something only younger people can operate. "If you can use a hand-held calculator, you can use a computer," he tells senior citizens. "Don't be afraid to give it a try. If you say you can't, you can't. If you say you can, you will."

Kathy Raffel

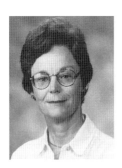

Kathy Raffel

For Mayo Clinic patient educator Kathy Raffel, tennis provides an opportunity to exercise her body and her mind at the same time. She took up the sport at the age of 42.

"In middle age, you have to approach tennis differently," says Raffel. Although middle-agers may not be as quick and strong as younger players, they can still be competitive by playing a mental game.

"At first, I focused on the physical game, smashing the ball to try to win, and coping with a sore body," explains Raffel. She soon realized she needed to work on her concentration and strategy, in addition to keeping physically fit.

Now she's a calmer, more strategic tennis player, focusing on improving her "mental toughness." With this competitive edge, she recently beat an agile 19-year-old.

"Starting the sport in middle age, I never thought I'd be on a team that would go to the nationals [competition]," Raffel says. Of course, you don't need to be competitive to enjoy the benefits of regular participation in sports.

Raffel plays tennis several times a week in a recreational league. In addition to the exercise, she values the team spirit and the social interaction.

"When I play tennis, my mind is cleared of day-to-day worries," says Raffel. "I love the game, and the challenge keeps me physically and mentally refreshed."

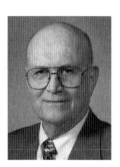

Dr. Fontana

Robert Fontana, M.D.

For the first 6 months of his retirement, Robert Fontana, M.D., woke up feeling restless and guilty. "I kept thinking to myself, 'I ought to be doing something,' and I think a lot of people feel that same way," he says.

For that reason, the retired pulmonologist joined the staff of the *Mayo Clinic Health Letter* on a part-time basis to answer some of the health questions sent in by readers. After working with the *Health Letter* for several years, Dr. Fontana recently turned his attention to evaluating the results of research studies on various aspects of lung disease.

Some people don't understand why he wants to continue working after retirement. Dr. Fontana's response is to tell them that he's the one who benefits from it.

"I retired from active practice, but I could never retire from medicine completely, " he admits. His involvement in research projects keeps him up-to-date on the ever-changing world of medicine.

"I think if you get away from challenging yourself regularly, it doesn't take long for you to go stale," he says. "I think that's true for anyone. Sitting around isn't good for your body or your mind."

Dr. Fontana encourages retirees to keep active, whether it's in the work world, doing volunteer activities or enjoying recreational pursuits.

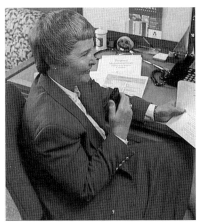

Dr. Audrey Nelson feels that goal-setting is crucial to meeting life's challenges.

Audrey M. Nelson, M.D.

"Always have a goal that you're working toward," advises rheumatologist Audrey M. Nelson, M.D.

Dr. Nelson takes that advice to heart for herself. During her career, she's had a series of goals that she set and achieved. As a senior consultant in rheumatology, Dr. Nelson is now beginning to set preliminary goals for her retirement.

"Retirement planning must be done well in advance and should be viewed as a transition from one career to another rather than an endpoint," Dr. Nelson says. She points out that individuals who have completed their primary careers have much to contribute to society in terms of their experience and talents. "They not only help other people, but broaden their own horizons in the process," she adds.

"People who have something to do have a better life," she says. "People who sit around are not as functional as they get older."

"Life is a series of steps," notes Dr. Nelson, "and you should always be looking for your next landing."

Make Your Health a Priority

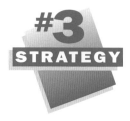

Make your health a priority. Simple as it may seem, it's one of the best, most practical choices you can make to lead a healthier and longer life, according to Mayo Clinic experts.

Your health depends a great deal on the responsibility you take for it. In many ways, you decide every day how healthy you're going to be. Not all diseases and conditions are avoidable, of course. But many of the most serious ones can be prevented by making good decisions each day about:

- Eating healthfully
- Maintaining a healthy weight
- Getting regular medical care
- Taking time to listen to your body

Making your health a priority doesn't mean giving up your favorite foods, activities or becoming concerned about your health to the exclusion of other things. It's about balance — making sure that taking care of yourself is as important as meeting your other responsibilities.

How you do this is up to you. But here's how these Mayo Clinic experts make their own health a priority.

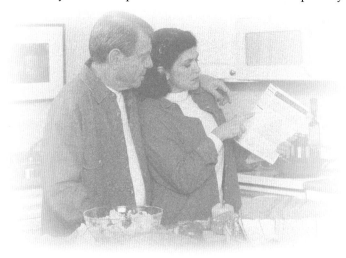

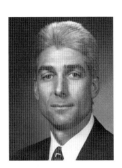

Dr. Hensrud

Donald Hensrud, M.D.

Making your health a priority doesn't have to be a matter of sacrifice, according to Donald Hensrud, M.D., a Mayo Clinic specialist in nutrition and endocrinology.

For example, Dr. Hensrud naturally makes healthy eating a part of his life — both at home and at work. But he still has an occasional passion for desserts that he's unwilling to give up.

"Are they the healthiest things in the world? No," he says. "But that's not the point. If I eat healthy 95 percent of the time, an occasional treat probably won't matter. To make your health a priority, you need to look at your lifestyle and make positive, not negative, changes."

For example, by working out with his wife each day on their home fitness equipment, exercise has become something he looks forward to and enjoys. "It keeps us and our marriage healthy," he says.

And when it comes to eating healthfully, Dr. Hensrud chooses to focus on the variety of healthy foods he can eat. He enjoys trying the new or exotic fruits and vegetables now available in produce sections. At home, he also makes sure that healthy foods are more visible and accessible to his family than less healthy ones.

"We're too caught up in focusing on restricting this and that, especially dietary fat," Dr. Hensrud says. "Although limiting some foods is important, there are plenty of great foods out there and you can learn to like new foods.

"Eating healthfully can mean eating well."

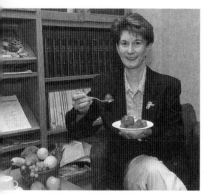

Jennifer Nelson follows her own advice about healthy eating.

Jennifer K. Nelson

As head of Mayo Clinic's dietetics department, Jennifer K. Nelson has helped thousands of people make healthier eating choices and understand the role nutrition plays in preventing disease. In the kitchen of her home in Rochester, Minnesota, she's worked to instill in her family the same appreciation of how much influence nutrition has on their health.

Lower-fat meals, attention to portion sizes and healthy cooking methods combine to makes meals at the Nelson household healthy ones. Inviting friends and family over for dinner makes meals enjoyable as well.

Nelson offers these tips for you, based on how she cooks for her family:

- You can reduce fat by up to half in almost any recipe without compromising flavor.
- Remember, the method of preparation is flexible. You don't need to fry food. Bake it, steam it or poach it. And let fat drip away during cooking.
- Emphasize whole grains and fresh fruits and vegetables. Filling up on these keeps higher-fat meats, dairy products and sweets in check.
- If you really must eat something high in fat or sugar, you can cut the size of the serving.

"Making your health a priority is something you don't have to do alone," Nelson says. "When you include your family and friends, it's easier to start and maintain healthy habits. And the nice thing is, you're helping others learn how to make choices that can help them lead healthier lives."

Philip Hagen, M.D.

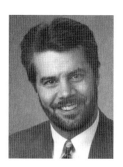

Dr. Hagen

As medical editor of the *Mayo Clinic Guide to Self-Care*, Philip Hagen, M.D., has literally written the book on making your health a priority. The book, which draws upon Dr. Hagen's experience as a specialist in preventive medicine, features practical advice on taking care of yourself and developing healthy habits.

For Dr. Hagen, the demands of being a physician along with responsibilities to his family and community can make practicing what he preaches difficult. Although he works hard to eat healthfully and get enough exercise, fitting everything in can be a challenge.

"The key is balance. You have to make sure your health doesn't take a back seat to 'the urgency of the moment' and everything else that's going on in your life," Dr. Hagen says.

To ensure this doesn't happen, Dr. Hagen makes it a point to analyze all aspects of his health a few times a year. He looks at four categories when evaluating his health:

Physical. "I ask myself: 'Am I eating a reasonably healthy diet? Am I getting enough rest? Am I getting exercise every day?'"

Dr. Hagen says you should think hard about your nutrition, your exercise habits, your health habits and keeping your immunizations up-to-date.

When was the last time you saw your doctor for preventive care? Dr. Hagen notes that you can determine the number of times you need a physical exam by decade, barring major medical problems. That means see your doctor two times when you're in your 20s, three times in your 30s, four times in your 40s and five times in your 50s. After 60, get an annual physical exam.

If you find that you've neglected your physical health, Dr. Hagen says don't panic, simply "make an adjustment."

Mental. Everybody needs at least one activity that's both challenging and enjoyable. Dr. Hagen coaches academic and sports teams and has served on several community development boards. But at each analysis, he makes sure that he's involved in a project that interests and challenges him.

Spiritual. For Dr. Hagen, spirituality means thinking seriously about one's place and purpose in the world. "Humans have a great need to have purpose in life," he says. "I fill this need through church, family discussions and reading."

Social support. Everyone needs supportive human contact to be healthy. Developing that social network should be a priority. At each analysis, Dr. Hagen makes sure his social life is healthy as well.

Birthdays, holidays and life changes offer good opportunities for self-analysis, Dr. Hagen says. "You can't afford to neglect any one category," he notes. "Like it or not, they all contribute to your health."

Don't Smoke

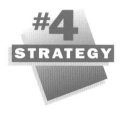

Another top strategy that's recommended by Mayo Clinic experts for a longer, healthier life should come as no surprise — don't smoke.

If you're a smoker, you're simply more likely to die early. Up to half of all current smokers will die of a disease caused by tobacco. Every year, at least 430,000 people in America die from the direct effects of smoking, and more than 50,000 nonsmokers die from the effects of secondhand smoke. Smoking leads to more deaths than AIDS, illegal drugs, alcohol, fire, automobile accidents, homicide and suicide combined.

And it's not just adults who are at risk. Children exposed to secondhand smoke are more likely to develop upper respiratory illnesses, asthma and ear infections. And maternal smoking before and after a baby's birth is a risk factor for sudden infant death syndrome (SIDS).

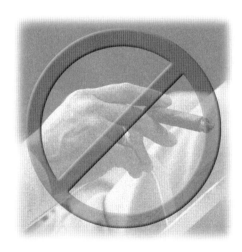

But there is good news. No matter what your age, if you stop smoking, you'll dramatically reduce your risk of disease, according to Richard D. Hurt, M.D., head of the Mayo Clinic Nicotine Dependence Center.

"It's never too late to stop," Dr. Hurt says. And he should know. See the next page for an account of his personal struggle with smoking and his ultimate success in kicking the habit.

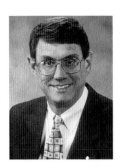

Dr. Hurt

Richard D. Hurt, M.D.

Through his work at the Mayo Nicotine Dependence Center, Dr. Hurt has helped thousands of smokers stop. But his knowledge of both the benefits and the difficulties of quitting come firsthand. Dr. Hurt is a former smoker who struggled to stop for many years.

"I smoked heavily right from the beginning and even smoked through medical school," he says. "I never met a cigarette I didn't like."

At one point, Dr. Hurt smoked two to three packs a day. As a physician, he knew the toll it was taking on his health. Although he stopped smoking dozens of times, he couldn't permanently break the grip that tobacco had on his life.

Then while a resident at Mayo Clinic, he enrolled in the Smokers' Clinic at Rochester Methodist Hospital, which offered support, information and understanding. With the program's help, Dr. Hurt finally stopped for good.

Years later, however, Dr. Hurt still remembers how hard it was going without a cigarette for the first time. "It was November 22, 1975. It was Saturday at 3:30 in the afternoon. I was home alone. It was the hardest thing I have ever done," he says.

Nicotine, the addictive drug in tobacco, can have serious withdrawal symptoms, and sometimes, they can last for months. Dr. Hurt himself experienced irritability, insomnia and nicotine cravings for weeks.

Fortunately, Dr. Hurt notes, today there are more treatment programs that have trained health care professionals to help smokers stop. Also, effective medications are available to ease cravings — including nicotine gum, nicotine patches, nicotine nasal spray, a nicotine inhaler and a non-nicotine medication.

But as helpful as these services and products are, Dr. Hurt says your success also depends on your commitment to stop smoking and do what's necessary to achieve your goal. Once you reach that point, he says, these tips can help:

- Ask your health care professional for help and advice on seeking out a formal treatment program.
- Set a date to stop smoking and stick to it. Make the date within the next 30 days.
- Plan to use at least one of the approved medications that help smokers stop.
- Think about what happened last time you tried to stop. Avoid places and activities that you connect with smoking, such as going to a bar or watching a lot of TV.
- Get rid of all your smoking paraphernalia.
- Don't try to smoke just one cigarette to ease your cravings. Most smokers can't stop at one.

Above all, be honest with yourself, Dr. Hurt says. "Quitting won't be easy, but the reasons for doing it far outweigh the reasons for continuing to smoke."

Invest in the Major Relationships in Your Life

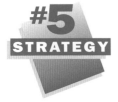

When it comes to your well-being, don't underestimate the importance of those closest to you. Whether it's your spouse, children or close friends, the people you count as family can play an important role in your health.

Strong relationships with your partner or family can motivate you to take care of yourself — to eat right, exercise and get regular medical care. Your partner and family can also be an important buffer from the stresses of everyday life. And if your health isn't good, your family may help get you the medical care you need or manage your condition more successfully.

But like a garden, family relationships need tending, according to Mayo Clinic experts. You can't expect to reap the benefits of long-term relationships unless you invest in them.

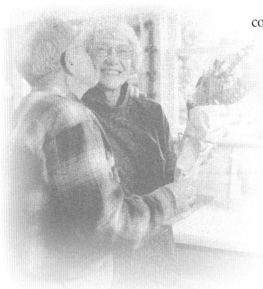

There is no right way to stay connected with your family. What's important is simply that you do it. Here's how these Mayo Clinic physicians invest in and benefit from the major relationships in their lives.

Andrew Good, M.D.

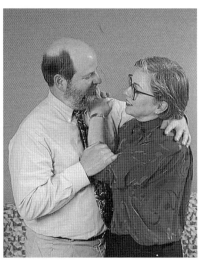

Dr. Andrew Good believes the secret to a longer, healthier life is a good relationship. He and his wife, Alison, have been married for 34 years.

The secret to a longer, healthier life, according to Andrew Good, M.D., is this: "Live with a loving partner in a relationship of mutual respect and sharing. It's easier for two to handle a problem than one."

Dr. Good bases his advice on personal experience. He and his wife, Alison, have been married for 34 years. In that time, they've raised two children and built a strong relationship in which each has grown and changed yet still maintained common ground.

For Dr. Good, sharing his life with Alison has been an important part of staying healthy — both physically and mentally. Talking with Alison and enjoying the comfortable companionship that comes with being partners for life plays a key role in helping Dr. Good relax and keep stress at bay. With Alison, he can share laughter, celebrate achievements or put problems in perspective.

Most importantly, Dr. Good says, his relationship with Alison keeps him looking forward to the years ahead. "With a life partner, you continue to grow, not just grow older, " he says.

Still, working at a relationship, even one as strong as his own, is critical, Dr. Good says. The couple regularly alternates bringing each other breakfast in bed. At home, dinners together are almost always by candlelight.

"The little things you can do to let the other person know they're special are important ways to invest in your relationship," Dr. Good says.

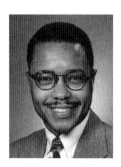

Dr. Willis

Floyd Willis, M.D.

As a family practice physician, Floyd Willis, M.D., estimates that stress plays a role in up to 40 percent of the diseases and conditions that bring patients to his office.

That's why Dr. Willis, who practices at Mayo Clinic's Jacksonville, Florida, location, makes spending time with his wife and two young children a top priority in his hectic schedule.

At home, mealtimes are a family occasion, where Dr. Willis and his family can catch up on the day's news. And whenever possible, he and his family head to the beaches to fish, build sand castles, or just enjoy the sights and sounds of the Atlantic Ocean.

"My family really helps me strike a balance," Dr. Willis says. "And when you do this, it has a positive effect on your physical and mental well-being."

Dr. Willis tells many of his patients that to stay healthy, it's not enough to simply have medical tests and report there's no problem. He advises people that the whole of life needs to be taken into account.

"You have to ask yourself if your lifestyle is healthy, too," he says. "If you're in tune with everything in your life, you're going to be much, much better off." Family is essential to "staying in tune," he adds.

He notes that your relationship with your partner can be an important foundation for helping you stay healthy and succeed in other areas of life. If you have children, building and keeping strong relationships can be a source of great joy — one that can help you keep your perspective if other things go wrong.

Even an extended family of relatives and friends can benefit you, Dr. Willis adds.

"Family can help nourish the soul," he says. "And for your health, that's as important to nourish as anything else."

Take Time for
the Things You Enjoy

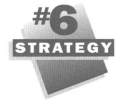

#6
STRATEGY

Do you enjoy gardening? Playing bridge? Traveling the globe? Spending time with your grandchildren?

You might be surprised to know that these activities not only bring enjoyment, but they also may benefit your health.

Science is only beginning to document the health benefits of leisure activities. But a growing number of studies suggest that taking time for the things you enjoy can help you feel better about yourself and more satisfied with life. And when you feel this way, you may be more likely to exercise, eat well, get regular medical care and reach out to friends and family — all of which can benefit you physically and mentally.

Not surprisingly, taking time for the things you enjoy is one of the prescriptions for a healthier, longer life that Mayo Clinic experts follow themselves.

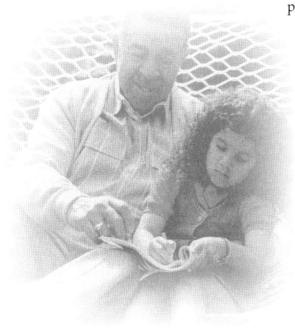

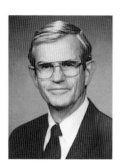

Dr. Lufkin

Here's how
they do it.

Edward Lufkin, M.D.

After practicing medicine for more than 30 years, Edward Lufkin, M.D., a former medical editor of the *Mayo Clinic Health Letter*, eagerly awaited the day he'd be fully retired and living in his lakeside cottage.

But Dr. Lufkin found that he wasn't quite ready to give up his medical lecturing. He signed a contract with a pharmaceutical company and now travels extensively, meeting with professional groups. "I enjoy the stimulation of travel and the medical world, but I also have plenty of time at the lake," he says.

He offers these thoughts about retirement in the cyber age:

- Take advantage of the many opportunities available through computers. You don't have to live near a shopping center to enjoy convenient shopping. You'll find almost any product on the Internet.
- Maintain contact with friends and family through e-mail. It's easy to learn — and you can do it in scruffy clothing!
- Explore the array of enjoyable games and discussion groups available through computers. Bridge, chess, solitaire, backgammon — almost all of the world's great games can be played on a computer.
- Don't stay glued to the TV. It can be a real time-taker if you let it. Getting a simple weather forecast can stretch out into an hour-long slouch in a chair.
- Take advantage of the dozens of Web sites available for health information. Check the source and the date to be sure it's recent and reputable.

Although the computer connects Dr. Lufkin and his family with the outside world, they treasure their home in the northern woods. "We have far closer contact with nature

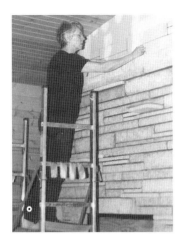

than city dwellers experience," he says, "and this is good for the soul."

Renée Bergstrom

Renée Bergstrom, a patient education specialist at Mayo Clinic, balances life by focusing on the process of creating beauty. Her artistic endeavors include gardening and photography, as well as designing and decorating her home and cottage.

She recently collaborated with her husband to construct a rock fireplace wall. "I sketched the pattern on the wall, two rows at a time, and my husband cut and positioned the pieces," she says.

Family and friends play a vital part in Bergstrom's life. With her camera, she's captured many tender and playful moments of her eight grand-children and their "BaPaw" (grandpa). Bergstrom uses her photographs of scenery to create postcards, bookmarks and posters for the Cornucopia Art Center in Lanesboro, Minnesota.

"Teaching stress management classes reminds me how important it is to keep balance in my life," she says. "I think everyone needs some type of creative outlet to handle the stresses of daily life."

Amazingly, she finds time to take classes in a doctoral program in education and leadership. "It's more for self-fulfillment and personal development than a definite career goal," says Bergstrom. "I believe in challenging my mind and have faith that I'll find or create ways to use my new skills."

Using her artistic talent, Renée Bergstrom works on her fireplace wall.

Mary Madden

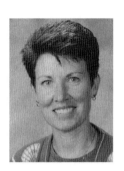

Mary Madden

Mary Madden, R.N., who works in obstetrics at Rochester Methodist Hospital, makes it a priority to take time for her favorite activities: reading, hiking and spending time outdoors with her family.

Hiking directly benefits Madden's health — the exercise increases her muscle strength and endurance. Over the years, she's taken in the beauty of the Minnesota state parks and nurtured the family bond by hiking with her husband and two sons.

"We recently hiked through national parks in Alaska, and the scenery is stunning," says Madden. "It's just you and the wilderness."

Books are especially important to Madden. Whether it's history, biographies or westerns, she's an avid reader of them all. "I make time to read — even if I have to sneak it in," she says. The books help her learn or fire her imagination, but the benefits go beyond this.

"For me, time devoted to reading and outdoor activities are the most effective stress management tools there are," she says. "They help me keep my balance. If

Do Pets Play a Role in Your Health?

A pet — whether it's a dog, cat, goldfish or iguana — can help you establish healthy habits or benefit your emotional health. For example, research shows that dog owners are more likely to walk regularly than people who don't

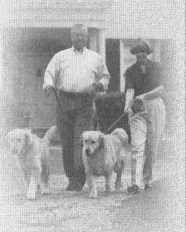

have dogs. Other research suggests that pet owners may feel less lonely or isolated, even if they live alone. Because social isolation is a powerful risk factor for poor health, having a pet may help you live longer and better.

Robert Sheeler, M.D. (see page 33), believes strongly in the healthy impact pets can have on your life. He currently has two cats: Gildor, who at 17 is always calm and even-tempered, and Finn, who is filled with youthful enthusiasm. "Having them around helps me unwind after a long day at work," he notes. In addition, the pets remind him and his wife to get outside and enjoy the outdoors.

"They remind you to live in the moment, and that the human perspective is but one of many ways to look at the world," Dr. Sheeler says.

Edward Creagan, M.D. (see page 7), a cancer specialist, also feels pets play an important role in his life. He has a dog and a cat. "These creatures can bring a tremendous sense of peace and tranquillity," he says.

Stay Connected to Your Community

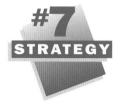

#7 STRATEGY

you have balance, you can get up in the morning and look forward to the new day."

Whether it's volunteering for a cause or simply befriending someone else, being part of a network of people can benefit you physically and mentally.

Research shows a link between quality of life and community involvement. It's only common sense. If you feel needed and a part of your community, you'll likely feel better about yourself and enjoy life more.

And staying connected to your community may also add years to your life. Science has only begun to document the effects of social support on your health. But a growing body of evidence suggests that staying connected with others can buffer or reduce some of the health-related effects of aging — or even extend your life.

In one study involving women 75 years old and older, researchers found that women with no friends or

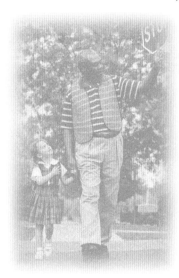

community ties were about twice as likely to die earlier than those with a social network. Other research suggests that older people who volunteer a moderate amount of their time may be more likely to live longer than those who don't. A social network may also play a role in helping you recover from a health condition.

Staying involved with your community can mean different things to different people. You may choose to volunteer with an organization, or you might participate in your church choir. Simply being involved is far more important than what you're involved in.

Here's how these Mayo Clinic experts stay involved in their communities.

Norman Hepper, M.D.

During his years of practice at Mayo Clinic, pulmonologist Norman Hepper, M.D., read medical charts, journals and thousands of X-rays.

In retirement, Dr. Hepper still devotes a great deal of time to reading. Only now, Dr. Hepper is being read to — by students at two elementary schools close to his home in Rochester, Minnesota.

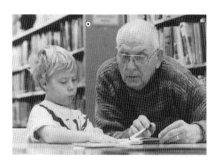

Dr. Norman Hepper listens intently as a young student reads aloud.
(Photo courtesy of Rochester *Post-Bulletin*)

As a volunteer in the schools' reading programs for the past 7 years, Dr. Hepper is as familiar to students as their teachers or principal. Each week, he spends time at the schools helping students sharpen their reading skills.

Working with each student individually, Dr. Hepper listens as the student reads aloud. When necessary, he helps the student pronounce a word or grasp a reading skill that's been difficult to understand.

"It's really a different world for me to be involved in, but it's very gratifying," Dr. Hepper says. "I feel like each school is my own. I know the teachers, the students and what they're doing. It's been very educational for me." A particular highlight, he notes, has been working with children from many different cultures.

Dr. Hepper is also involved in other community activities. Between volunteering and activities with friends, he's rarely home for lunch. But he wouldn't have it any other way.

Community involvement, he says, has widened his circle of friends and given him a sense of fulfillment that he wouldn't have found otherwise. "Community

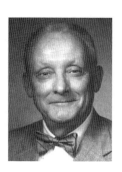

Dr. Kiely

involvement is so important," he says. "And it's something anybody can do."

Joseph Kiely, M.D.

Joseph Kiely, M.D., believes he's part of a global community. In that spirit, the retired hematologist spends a month each year helping others in a place far from the peaceful, rolling hills that surround Mayo Clinic.

Every January, Dr. Kiely travels to Haiti and sets up practice in a clinic and hospital in a remote village. There, underneath the bright Caribbean sunshine, he puts the skills honed at Mayo Clinic to use treating people who normally have little access to medical care.

The weather is hot, the hours are long and the political climate unstable, but Dr. Kiely doesn't mind. Tending those who come to the clinic makes him feel needed and "part of the solution, not the problem."

"These trips are an opportunity to give something back," he says. "And actually, the experience is so positive that I get more out of it than I give."

Dr. Kiely, the founding medical editor of the *Mayo Clinic Health Letter*, believes this is true for many reasons. For one, his research into the diseases he encounters in Haiti (many of them have virtually disappeared in the United States) keeps him sharp. He's also able to connect with many different and interesting people when they come to work at the clinic. In addition, his work there reminds him how privileged his life has been and continues to be.

That, he says, is enough to keep him thinking positively a long time after he returns to Minnesota.

Dr. Kiely urges others, especially older people, to get involved in their communities in any way possible. "No matter how old you are, you can still be

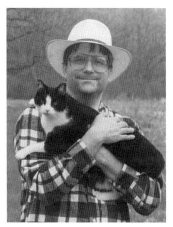

Dr. Robert Sheeler poses with "Gil." (See "Do pets play a role in your health?" on page 29.)

very helpful and useful. And feeling that way makes you feel better yourself."

Robert Sheeler, M.D.

Volunteering isn't the only way to stay connected to your community. You can also find others with whom to share hobbies or interests, as Robert Sheeler, M.D., has done.

In addition to being a family practice specialist and medical editor of the *Mayo Clinic Health Letter*, Dr. Sheeler enjoys reading. Through this interest, both he and his wife, Pat, stay connected with friends and the community around them.

Dr. Sheeler and his wife are part of the Diverse Readers Book Club, an informal gathering of friends and acquaintances that meets regularly to debate and discuss books from an assigned reading list.

Books covered by the group include everything from mysteries to works by noted writers. Not only is the reading list diverse, so is the group. Members include computer programmers, engineers, lawyers and bookstore employees.

"It's really inspiring and thought provoking," Dr. Sheeler says. "Everyone has such different backgrounds and philosophies."

Although the discussion is challenging, Dr. Sheeler notes that an important benefit of the book club is seeing other members and getting to know them. He believes that this feeling of being connected to a larger group helps both him and his wife feel and stay healthier.

"The relationships you have with your family and the community around you are important," he says. "Building both types of ties is an enjoyable and worthwhile investment in your health."

GLOSSARY

Dementia: Mental deterioration due to organic causes.

Endocrinology: Pertains to the endocrine system, which is comprised of the glands that function as a control system for the human body. Diabetes and thyroid disorders are examples of common endocrine conditions.

Hematologist: A doctor who specializes in diseases of the blood and blood-forming organs.

Immunizations: Introductions of antigens (substances foreign to the body that cause antibodies to form) in very small quantities in order to stimulate the development of immunity.

Osteoarthritis: A joint disorder known as the "wear-and-tear arthritis," which is caused by a deterioration of cartilage in a joint.

Osteoporosis: A bone-weakening disease caused by a gradual loss of calcium and other minerals from bones, making them thinner, weaker and prone to fracture.

Pulmonologist: A doctor who specializes in diseases of the lungs.

Rheumatologist: A doctor who specializes in joint and muscle diseases caused by abnormalities in the immune system and degradation of the joints, as well as inflammation of arteries.

Sudden infant death syndrome: The sudden and unexplained death of an apparently healthy infant.